Rim Khemakhem
Donia Ben Jmeaa

Long-COVID syndrome

Rim Khemakhem
Donia Ben Jmeaa

Long-COVID syndrome

Understanding Symptoms and Predictive Factors

ScienciaScripts

Imprint

Cover image: www.ingimage.com

This book is a translation from the original published under ISBN 978-620-3-45825-1.

Publisher:
Sciencia Scripts
is a trademark of
Dodo Books Indian Ocean Ltd. and OmniScriptum S.R.L publishing group

120 High Road, East Finchley, London, N2 9ED, United Kingdom
Str. Armeneasca 28/1, office 1, Chisinau MD-2012, Republic of Moldova, Europe
Managing Directors: Ieva Konstantinova, Victoria Ursu
info@omniscriptum.com

Printed at: see last page
ISBN: 978-620-8-53745-6

PLAN

INTRODUCTION

Coronavirus 2019 (COVID-19) is a contagious infectious disease caused by severe acute respiratory syndrome coronavirus 2 (SARS-CoV-2). This is an enveloped RNA virus transmitted mainly by respiratory droplets (1).The first known case of COVID-19 was identified in Wuhan, China, in December 2019. In March 2020, the World Health Organisation (WHO) declared the COVID-19 epidemic a pandemic, due to its rapid transmission and high hospitalisation and mortality rates. The main modes of transmission included respiratory droplets and direct or indirect contact with contaminated surfaces. The COVID-19 pandemic, caused by the SARS-CoV-2 virus, had a profound impact on the early 2020s, affecting almost every aspect of global society. The pandemic caused millions of deaths worldwide, mainly affecting the elderly and those with co-morbidities such as diabetes or cardiovascular disease. Hospitals were often overwhelmed, lacking beds, respirators and nursing staff. The rapid development of vaccines represented a major scientific advance.According to the WHO update of 18 December 2023, 772,386,069 people have been infected with COVID-19 worldwide, with 6,987,222 deaths (2). Tunisia was one of the worst affected countries, with 115,3361 people infected and 29,423 deaths (2.6%) (2). In the early stages of the COVID-19 pandemic, it was recognised that the effects of SARS-CoV-2 were likely to vary from asymptomatic infection to multi-systemic disease. COVID-19 is therefore a complex disease, involving viral, inflammatory and thrombotic phases (1). To this day, the enormous concern raised by the SARS-CoV- 2 pandemic in terms of public health management social impact is still the subject of much debate. debate, particularly because COVID-19 can affect people infected for much longer than expected by a typical airborne viral disease (3-6). Indeed, COVID-19 can have long-lasting consequences, well beyond the acute phase infection. According to the WHO, around 10% to 20% of these people experience various medium- and long-term effects after the initial recovery (7). These symptoms may have persisted since the onset of the disease or they may appear after the initial recovery. They may be intermittent or reappear after a period of time (7).The most common symptoms associated with post-COVID-19 are breathlessness, general weakness, muscle pain, cognitive dysfunction, headaches, loss of smell, hair loss, nausea and vomiting, all of which affect the quality of life of those affected (3-7).These signs and symptoms were finally described as "long COVID", the most widespread definition of which is "new signs and symptoms occurring 4 to 8 weeks after the end of the acute phase of COVID-19" and cannot be explained by an alternative diagnosis. (8). Symptoms may also fluctuate or recur over time. Long COVID is therefore not a simple disease, but a complex disorder due to the dysfunction of several organ systems; it is therefore probably more appropriate to speak of a syndrome (9,10). In the majority of people infected with SARS-CoV-2, the live virus is completely eliminated within days or weeks of infection and is no longer detectable in the respiratory system. However, clearance of viral RNA or antigen from respiratory epithelia or other tissue sites may be slow and, in some cases, viruses may persist in forms that are not well understood. Fundamental questions about the relationship between the persistence of SARS-CoV-2 and the longevity of the symptoms of long COVID have not been resolved (11).For this reason, research into the risk factors associated with the development of long COVID is highlighted as a necessity (12). It is therefore important to continue to study and understand the long-term implications of COVID-19 in order to develop appropriate management and treatment approaches, as well as prevention strategies.

CHAPTER I

EPIDEMIOLOGICAL DATA

1. Frequency of long covid

Long COVID, also known as post-acute sequelae of SARS-CoV-2 infection, refers to a series of persistent or recurrent symptoms that occur in some people after the acute phase of COVID-19 infection. This phenomenon has been recognised as a significant medical problem since patients have reported long-lasting symptoms even months after their initial recovery. Long COVID can seriously alter the daily lives of those affected:

- Inability to work or resume a normal life.

- Social isolation due to fatigue or physical limitations.

- Emotional and mental disorders linked to persistent symptoms.

This is a diagnosis exclusion, which means that doctors must first rule out other possible causes of the symptoms. It is based on :

- A thorough clinical assessment.

• Additional tests (imaging, blood tests) to identify any specific complications.

The frequency of patients presenting with long covid syndrome varied from one study to another, ranging from 22% to 63% (13-15). An Italian study (16) found that 87% of recovered patients had at least one persistent symptom after 60 days.

This difference in the results of the various studies could be explained by the difference in the populations studied, the way in which they are measured, the SARS-CoV-2 variant and the vaccination status. This is why the exact prevalence of post-covid syndrome cannot be estimated (17).

2. Age

Although Long Covid can affect people of any age, the experience of the disease varies according to age, co-morbidities and personal circumstances. The average age of patients with long Covid syndrome is around 50 [40-60 years] (18-20). Younger adults may also be affected, but they often report different or symptoms. Indeed, some studies have found a younger average age between 36 and 39 years

(15,21).In adults of working age, long COVID can have a significant economic and social impact, leading to an inability to work or a reduction in productivity. So a personalised approach remains the key to effectively managing its impact.

3. Gender

Most of the data in the literature have noted a female predominance (16, 22 24), with the exception of a few studies (18). The female predominance of post-covid syndrome found in the literature could be explained by the fact that female hormones may play a role in perpetuating the inflammatory state of the acute phase of SARS-CoV-2 infection even after recovery. Indeed, a higher production of Immunoglobulin G (IgG) antibodies in women at the onset of the disease was reported, which could result in a more favourable outcome in women, but could also play a role in perpetuating the manifestations of the disease. In addition, it could be hypothesised that women are generally more attentive to their bodies and the distress associated with them (25,26).

As women are often the main carers in households, they may be more exposed to the virus and report more symptoms because of their active role in managing their own health and that of their loved ones. These differences highlight the importance of taking gender into account diagnosis, research and care management for patients with long-standing COVID.

A personalised approach and greater recognition of these disparities could significantly improve patient care. Care must be tailored to the specific needs of patients, depending on their gender, symptoms and medical history.

4. Vaccination

Vaccination has been a decisive turning point in the fight against COVID-19. Although it does not guarantee absolute protection against infection, it remains an essential tool for preventing severe forms of the disease and controlling the impact of the pandemic. Several types of vaccine against COVID-19 have been developed rapidly as a result of global research efforts. Vaccination against COVID-19 was a major breakthrough in the fight against the pandemic caused by SARS-CoV-2. It has led to a significant reduction in severe forms of the disease, hospital admissions and deaths, and has facilitated the resumption of social and economic activities. The relationship between COVID-19 vaccination and long COVID has the subject of numerous studies since the start of the pandemic. Studies carried out in Bangladesh, Pakistan, Nepal and India have shown vaccination percentages equal to 20.6%, 22.1%, 26.2% and 28.1% respectively (27).

A cross-sectional study (26) conducted in February 2022 among Tunisian individuals infected with COVID-19 between March 2020 and February 2022 showed that 73.2% of participants were unvaccinated, 7.7% partially vaccinated and 19.1% had a complete vaccination schedulc against COVID-19.

In fact, the percentage of subjects with a complete vaccination schedule varies from one country to another, ranging from 8.2% in Afghanistan to 72.6% in Bhutan (27).

CHAPTER II

CLINICAL AND PARACLINICAL DATA

1. Signs lung

The pulmonary symptoms of long COVID are varied and can significantly impair quality of life. Regular medical monitoring and appropriate treatment are essential to improve respiratory function and prevent complications.

Given that the SARS-CoV-2 virus has a predominantly respiratory tropism, respiratory symptoms (dyspnoea and to a lesser extent dry cough) were at the forefront of the signs of post-covid syndrome (28-30). The pulmonary signs of long COVID are frequent in people who have had an initial severe or moderate infection with SARS-CoV-2, but can also appear after mild forms. Indeed, several studies have shown that the persistence of respiratory symptoms, particularly dyspnoea and cough, beyond 4 weeks after their onset, is frequent.

A multicentre observational cohort study of 1250 COVID-19 survivors in Michigan, USA (31), found that 15.4% of subjects who responded to the telephone survey reported the onset or worsening of a cough 2 months after the initial diagnosis.

A meta-analysis by Alkodaymi et al (32) showed that despite the heterogeneity of the studies, the frequency of dyspnoea approximately 25% between 3 and 6 months and 31% at 12 months follow-up.

Mendola M et al (33) found that exertional dyspnoea was the most frequent symptom 12 months after COVID-19 infection.

A study (34) followed patients previously admitted to respiratory units for acute respiratory failure secondary to COVID-19 pneumonia, 1 year after discharge. Pulmonary function tests (spirometry, carbon monoxide diffusion capacity (DLCO)) were used to assess lung volumes and carbon monoxide diffusion capacity. carbon dioxide (CO 2). Three out of thirty-three patients (9%) had an FEV1/FVC < 0.70 and 6 patients (18%) had an FVC less than 80%. In total, almost half of the patients (16/33, 49%) showed a reduction in DLCO.

Covid-19 infection, primarily causing acute respiratory distress, may be responsible for significant endothelial damage and an intense immune and inflammatory response in the lungs and airways via SARS-CoV-2 replication within endothelial cells (29). Song et al (35) have suggested that neurological, inflammatory and immunomodulatory pathways via the sensory nerves of the vagus nerve may contribute to cough hypersensitivity. More specifically, a post-viral neuropathy of the vagus nerve could play a role, involving both the sensory and motor branches of this nerve.

Sensation in the larynx is mediated in part by the superior laryngeal nerve, which also innervates the cricothyroid muscle. Dysfunction of this nerve can lead to various symptoms associated with chronic coughing and abnormal sensations in the laryngeal region, such as globus pharyngis (a feeling of a lump in the throat), throat clearing or a tickling sensation.

Chest CT plays a crucial role in the diagnosis and follow-up of patients with COVID-19 pneumonia.

A study including 114 patients of whom 40 (35%), who recovered from covid-19 pneumonia, fibrotic-like changes within 6 months (36). Another study (37), comparing CT images during and after the acute phase of SARS-CoV-2 infection, showed that lesions were significantly reduced and lesion density decreased. Indeed, CT lesions were completely resorbed in 64.7% of patients after 4 weeks (37). This indicates that the damage caused to lung tissue by COVID-19 may be reversible. Post-COVID-19 pulmonary fibrosis is the main irreversible lesion. It is accompanied by various lesions, such as interstitial abnormalities including cross-linking, traction bronchiectasis and ray-of-mine lesions (28). Histologically, it corresponds to a pathological reconstruction of the alveolar epithelium with an overproduction of collagenous extracellular matrix associated with a destruction of the normal pulmonary architecture (28).

2. Cardiovascular signs

Long COVID can have a significant impact on the cardiovascular system, leading to a variety of cardiovascular signs and symptoms. Palpitations and chest pain were the most frequent cardiovascular signs (30, 38, 39). Indeed, Chilazi et al (38) found the presence of chest pain and palpitations in 20% and 14% of subjects respectively 60 days acute infection with covid-19. In a study by Davis et al (40) involving 3,762 patients, more than half the subjects had chest pain (~ 53%) and palpitations (~ 68%) at 7 months after the acute infection. On the other hand, other studies have found lower percentages of no more than 11% (20, 41). The cardiovascular signs of long COVID may be multifactorial, involving inflammatory processes, direct tissue damage caused by the virus, disturbances to the autonomic nervous system immune responses (30, 38).

Numerous studies have suggested a correlation between long Covid syndrome and postural orthostatic tachycardia syndrome (POTS), a form of dysautonomia found in 10% to 41% of patients with post-covid syndrome (42). POTS is characterised by an excessive increase in heart rate when moving from lying to standing, which can lead to symptoms such as palpitations, chest pain, dizziness and a feeling of weakness (42).

A study carried out in Tunisia (43), including 618 patients, suggested that the alteration of the Left Ventricular Longitudinal Global Strain after COVID- 19 infection could be linked to endothelial dysfunction, which can be caused by different factors such as inflammation of cardiomyocytes, hypoxia and myocardial injury due to microvascular dysfunction. This alteration could contribute to the persistent chest pain observed in some patients after infection with COVID-19.

3. Signs neurological

Several studies have reported that headache is a frequent neurological symptom following infection with COVID-19 (16, 44, 45).

A cross-sectional study conducted in February 2022 and including

Tunisian patients infected with COVID-19 between March 2020 and February 2022 (26) revealed the presence of neurological symptoms in 36.6% of patients, including memory disorders (49.1%) and headaches (31.8%).

Furthermore, neuropathic pain, which may be a symptom in the acute phase of COVID-19, is more frequent in the context of long covid syndrome (46).

These neurological symptoms of long Covid have a negative impact on patients' quality of life, particularly in the case of impaired concentration, confusion and mental fatigue (47,48).

The GeroCovid Acute Wards study (48) showed that more than a fifth of patients lost at least one activity of daily living, the most common being bathing, dressing and transferring, probably due to increased difficulty in performing tasks requiring balance and coordination.

Persistent neurological signs remote from acute infection with covid-19 could be linked to the presence of SARS-CoV 2 in the cerebrospinal fluid (CSF), reflecting its neuroinvasive characteristics (16). In addition, it has been shown that there is a possible disruption of the microstructural and functional integrity of the brain in patients who have been infected COVID-19 (16).

SARS-CoV-2 enters human cells by binding to the angiotensin-converting enzyme 2 (ACE2) receptor. This receptor is known to be highly expressed not only in the lower respiratory tract, but also in certain parts of the brain, notably areas of the cortex. somatosensory, rectal/orbital gyrus, temporal lobe, hypothalamus/thalamus, brainstem and cerebellum. Direct viral infection of neuronal cells in these regions occurs when the virus binds to the ACE2 receptor and disrupts the blood-brain barrier. This invasion causes organic changes in the cells such as demyelination/neurodegeneration and reduced metabolic activity due to mitochondrial dysregulation. Some researchers have suggested that SARS-CoV2 is latent in neurons, leading to demyelination and neurodegeneration and a higher risk of long-term effects in some patients (47).

The prolonged immune response due to COVID-19 and the effects of cytokine storms are also possible mechanisms responsible for the neuropsychiatric symptoms of long covid. Inflammation of cerebral blood vessels leads to destruction of the blood-brain barrier and infiltration of immune cells into brain cells. In fact, studies have reported signs of reactive astrogliosis in the post-mortem tissues of COVID-19 patients, in cell models and in brain organoids. Indeed, studies using cerebral positron emission tomography (PET) in patients with long-standing COVID have revealed the presence of hypometabolism in certain regions of the brain in these patients, which may be linked to astroglial inflammation (47, 49).

In addition, systemic inflammation, including that of blood vessels throughout the body, can contribute to the development of persistent systemic symptoms, which in turn can lead to neuropsychiatric symptoms (47).

Another study including 785 participants, studying brain structure and cognitive function before the pandemic, was used to assess the effects of COVID-19. Neuropsychological and magnetic resonance imaging (MRI) data were used to compare participants testing positive for COVID-19 to those who remained unaffected. A second evaluation, including MRI, was carried out on average 38 months after the first. The authors found a reduction in grey matter in patients with COVID-19, particularly in the orbitofrontal cortex and parahippocampal gyrus. White matter changes were also observed in survivors, suggesting axonal alterations that could explain the persistence of headaches, but the specificity of these changes remains to be determined (50).

4. Otorhinolaryngological signs

Most of the studies published at the start of the pandemic suggested that most patients recovered normal odour function after a short period of infection with COVID-19 (51,52).

Reiter et al (51) reported that 72% of patients recovered from olfactory dysfunction (OD) within 1 month on the basis of anamnestic assessment. Niklaasen et al (52) reported that most people affected by covid-19 recovered 28 days, but that approximately 27% were still suffering from various degrees of OD after 28 to 169 days from the onset of symptomatology.

Another study (53) including 102 patients who underwent chemosensory testing 111 to 457 days after the onset of OD and taste dysfunction caused by COVID-19, found that 72.5% of patients had hyposmia, 4% had anosmia and 18.6% of patients had hypogueusia.

Other studies (19,44, 54,55) have also shown that the percentage of ENT disorders reached even more than 30% and that more than 15 million people worldwide suffered from persistent olfactory dysfunction due to covid- 19. The ENT symptoms could be explained by the fact that the SARS-CoV- 2 virus has a neurological tropism for both the central nervous system (CNS) and the peripheral nervous system (PNS).Given that ACE2 receptors expressed in the PNS may also be expressed in supporting neuronal cells associated with the taste and smell complex, this raises the possibility of direct damage to the PNS by COVID-19 leading to a state of chronic inflammation directly affecting the taste and smell system and viral invasion of the olfactory bulb. triggering a cascade of degeneration similar to Alzheimer's disease and Lewy body disease, which is a possible explanation for the development and maintenance of the long-term taste impairment associated with COVID-19 (19, 55,56).

Another possible mechanism of taste dysfunction involves the functional link taste and smell, whereby taste perception is reduced due to anterior olfactory sensory dysfunction (57).

5. Signs psychiatric

Using self-report questionnaires, several studies have found a high prevalence of insomnia (31-54%), anxiety (5-46%), depressive symptoms (9-42%) and post-traumatic stress symptoms (10-57%) (16,20, 28,47, 58). The COVID-19 Metabolic and Brain Consequences (COMEBAC) study reported insomnia in 54% of patients, anxiety symptoms in 31%, depressive symptoms in 22% and post-traumatic stress symptoms in 14% of patients 4 months after infection with COVID-19 (59).

Janiri et al (60) reported the onset of a new mental disorder within 3 months of the acute episode in 12% of patients. Another study by Mazza et al (61) reported that the prevalence of post-traumatic stress disorder was 30% 1 to 3 months after a severe acute episode.

A multicentre study carried out in Spain on 1,142 patients, 7 months after the initial phase of COVID-19 infection, showed that 34.5% them had poor sleep quality (62). The prevalence of depression and anxiety was 19.7% (HADS-depression ≥ 10 points) and 16.2% (HADS-anxiety ≥ 12 points) respectively (62).However, the frequency of sleep disorders varied between studies, ranging from 18% to 34% (62, 63).

The anxiety-provoking social and media context, the fear of a serious form of the disease, the fear of not being able to benefit from appropriate care, particularly in the first few weeks of the pandemic, the absence of an established cure, the lack of visits from family and friends following hospitalisation or because of confinement, and the traumatic experiences of the acute illness and care, sometimes in poor conditions, may have encouraged the onset of post-traumatic stress. Finally, the persistence of physical problems for weeks or months after the acute episode may have contributed to psychological symptoms and sleep disorders (28).In addition, the presence of SARS-CoV-2 in cerebrospinal fluid (CSF) demonstrates its neuroinvasive characteristics, and there is a possible disruption of the microstructural and functional integrity of the brain in patients recovered from COVID-19 (16).

6. Fatigue

According to the literature, 63% of patients still had a chronic fatigue problem 6 months after infection with SARS-CoV-2 (14-15, 20, 21, 29, 44).Several factors may play a role in the development of post-COVID-19 fatigue. Ortelli et al (64) have shown that interleukin-6-related hyperinflammation may play a role in central neuromotor and cognitive fatigue, apathy and executive/motivational dysfunction in long COVID by negatively regulating gamma-aminobutyric acid (GABA) receptors.In addition, negative psychological and social factors associated with the COVID-19 pandemic have also been linked to chronic fatigue. In addition, direct SARS-CoV-2 infection of skeletal muscle, causing muscle damage and weakness, may contribute to fatigue (65).

7. Pain joints

Several studies have noted the presence of joint pain remote from the acute episode of Covid-19 infection in approximately one-fifth of the patients studied (66-68).Joint pain is mainly caused by local pathological changes. Nociceptors are triggered by both mechanical and chemical stimuli, in particular pro-inflammatory factors, which could explain the mechanism of joint pain (69).

CHAPTER III

FACTORS PREDICTIVE OF LONG COVID

The data in the literature show that advanced age is a predictive factor for having a long covid (13, 16, 26, 57, 70, 71). Chelly et al also found that women had a higher risk having a long covid (57).

Some studies have not found a statistically significant association with diabetes, hypertension, obesity, severe disease in the acute phase and the delta variant compared with the omicron variant (57, 70). However, a study carried out in India (72) found a significant association between diabetes, arterial hypertension and long covid. Some studies have found that increased and prolonged inflammation, defective adaptive immune responses, endothelial dysfunction and coagulation-related disorders are phenomena well described in obesity and could represent a plausible explanation for the link high body mass index (BMI) and long covid (57, 70).Furthermore, the data in the literature concerning the association between the severity of the initial viral infection and residual symptoms are contradictory (13, 15, 24).

A study by magnusson et al (73) of 323,145 Norwegian adults showed that the risk of developing symptoms of covid was almost equivalent in those recovering from sars-cov- 2 omicron and delta. However, in another study (74), antonelli et al followed nearly 56,000 adults in the united Kingdom infected with sars-cov-2 between december 2021 and march 2022 and concluded that the risk of long-lasting covid was consistently lower in patients with sars-cov-2 omicron than in those with the delta variant.

1. Predictors of respiratory symptoms in Covid- long

Given that covid infection is mainly respiratory and that dyspnoea and dry cough were the most frequent signs of long covid, a correlation was between these two clinical signs and a history of asthma, COPD, SAS and smoking. Asthmatic patients had a higher risk of dry cough and post-covid dyspnoea than non-asthmatic patients (53, 75, 76). This could be explained by mast cell activation syndrome and the biased Th-2 immunological response (25).

A study by Chen Y et al showed that smoking increases the risk of dry cough following acute infection with covid 19 by 6.95 times (77).

Similarly, another retrospective cross-sectional study carried out in Bangladesh showed that a history of COPD and smoking were risk factors for persistent dyspnoea 2 months after recovery from covid-19 (78). A multicentre observational cohort study of 1250 COVID-19 survivors in Michigan, USA, showed that the persistence a dry cough after the initial diagnosis of covid-19 did not correlate with the degree of severity of the acute episode of infection (31).

2. Predictors of cardiovascular symptoms in Covid long

Female gender and hospitalisation during the acute phase of infection were risk factors for palpitations at a distance from the acute episode of infection according to the study by Brigido et al (54). However, Golchin Vafa et al (30) found no association between these two risk factors and long-standing palpitations. They also found that hospitalisation was a risk factor for chest pain following acute covid-19 infection.

3. Factors predictive of neurological signs of covid- long

Female gender was a risk factor for post-COVID headache (42, 50, 79). Studies have shown that female gender and the initial severity of the infection are risk factors for memory disorders in the long covid (29, 47). On the other hand, neuropathic pain was correlated with length of hospitalisation in some studies (80). Loss of autonomy, reported as a sign of post-covid syndrome, was associated with advanced age in a prospective study (81) conducted from May 2020 to

December 2021 involving 1,024 Polish people with a history of SARS-CoV-2 infection, which showed that older people had a greater risk of loss of autonomy.

4. Factors predictive of ENT symptoms in long- covid

Studies have considered the female sex as a risk factor for agueusia in the long covid (53, 57). Similarly, according to some authors, this risk factor plays a role in the development of anosmia in long covid (47, 53, 57).

5. Predictive factors for psychological disorders of the long-covid

Depression was correlated hospitalisation in a systematic review and meta-analysis by Badenoch et al (82). In addition, female gender and a history of COPD were risk factors for anxiety in the literature (47, 81).

Some authors have found that female gender, diabetes, obesity and arterial hypertension were predictive factors of sleep disorders in long covid (47).

6. Factors predictive of fatigue during long- covid

The female sex is considered to be a risk factor for fatigue (14, 20, 22, 53, 81, 83). On the other hand, some studies have noted that advanced age is a risk factor long covid fatigue (24, 84).

7. Factors predictive of joint pain in covid- long

Joint pain is a symptom frequently reported by people suffering Covid long, a condition that persists long after the acute phase of SARS-CoV-2 infection. This pain, often referred to as arthralgia (joint pain without inflammation), can affect various parts of the body and impair quality of life. Studies are underway to better understand the mechanisms of Covid long, in particular its link with musculoskeletal pain, and the most effective treatments. According to the literature, the female sex is a risk factor for long covid joint pain (24,29,69,81, 85).

CONCLUSION

Coronavirus 2019 (COVID-19) is a contagious infectious disease caused by the severe acute respiratory syndrome coronavirus 2 (SARS-CoV-2). COVID-19 can have lasting consequences, well beyond the acute phase infection. These signs and symptoms have been described as "long COVID".

Long COVID manifests itself through a variety of symptoms affecting several organ systems, making it complex to diagnose and manage. It therefore represents a challenge for healthcare systems because of its long-term implications for healthcare resources and services.

The most common symptoms associated with post-COVID-19 found in the literature are shortness of breath, general weakness, muscle pain, cognitive dysfunction, headache, loss of sense of smell, nausea and vomiting, all of which affect the quality of life of those affected.

Fundamental questions concerning the relationship between the persistence of SARS- CoV-2 and the longevity of symptoms of long-onset COVID remain unresolved. As a result, research into the risk factors associated with the development of long-onset COVID is highlighted as a necessity.

And although progress has been made in understanding long covid, much remains to be learned about the condition. Further research, increased awareness and coordinated management efforts are needed to meet the needs of patients with long-onset covid and mitigate its impact on public health.

BIBLIOGRAPHY

1. Bonny V, Maillard A, Mousseaux C, Plaçais L, Richier Q. COVID-19: pathophysiology of a multifaceted disease. Rev de Médecine Interne. 1 June 2020;41(6):375 89.

2. World Health Organization. COVID-19 cases. WHO COVID-19 dashboard. Dec 2023;1-13.

3. Camerlingo C. Post COVID syndrome: a new challenge for medicine. European Review. 2021;25(12):4422-4425.

4. Haute Autorité de Santé. Prolonged symptoms following adult Covid-19. Diagnosis and management. HAS. Jan 2023;1-11.

5. National Institutes of . COVID-19 Research. Long COVID. NIH. Sept 2023;1-6.

6. Chippa V, Aleem A, Anjum F. Post-Acute Coronavirus (COVID-19) Syndrome. Treasure Island (FL): StatPearls Publishing. 2023;NBK570608:1-2.

7. World Health Organisation. Coronavirus disease (COVID-19): post-COVID-19 condition. WHO. March 2023;1-5.

8. Regunath H, Goldstein NM, Guntur VP. Long COVID: Where Are

We in 2023. Mo Med. 2023;120(2):102 5.

9. Word Health Organization: A clinical case definition of post COVID-19 condition by a Delphi consensus. WHO. Oct 2021;1-27.

10. Szabo S, Zayachkivska O, Hussain A, Muller V. What is really "Long COVID"? Inflammopharmacology. Apr 2023;31(2):551 7.

11. Chen B, Julg B, Mohandas S, Bradfute SB. Viral persistence, reactivation, and mechanisms of long COVID. eLife. 2023;12:e86015.

12. Subramanian A, Nirantharakumar K, Hughes S, Myles P, Williams T, Gokhale KM, et al. Symptoms and risk factors for long COVID in non-hospitalized adults. Nat Med. 2022;28(8):1706 14.

13. Lippi G, Sanchis-Gomar F, Henry BM. COVID-19 and its long-term sequelae: what do we know in 2023? Pol Arch Intern Med. 19 Apr 2023;133(4):16402.

14. Fatima S, Ismail M, Ejaz T, Shah Z, Fatima S, Shahzaib M, et al. Association between long COVID and vaccination: A 12 month follow-up study in a low- to middle-income country. PLoS One. 22 Nov 2023;18(11):e0294780.

15. Arjun MC, Singh AK, Pal D, Das K, G. A, Venkateshan M, et al. Characteristics and predictors of Long COVID among diagnosed

cases of COVID-19. PLOS ONE. 20 Dec 2022;17(12):e0278825.

16. Raveendran AV, Jayadevan R, Sashidharan S. Long COVID: An overview. Diabetes & Metabolic Syndrome. June 2021;15(3):869.

17. Singh SJ, Baldwin MM, Daynes E, Evans RA, Greening NJ, Jenkins RG, et al. Respiratory sequelae of COVID-19: pulmonary and extrapulmonary origins, and approaches to clinical care and rehabilitation. Lancet Respir Med. 2023;11(8):709-725.

18. Squillace N, Cogliandro V, Rossi E, Bellelli G, Pozzi M, Luppi F, et al. A multidisciplinary approach to screen the post-COVID-19 conditions. BMC Infect Dis. 24 Jan 2023;23(1):54.

19. García-Vicente P, Rodríguez-Valiente A, Górriz Gil C, Márquez Altemir R, Martínez-Pérez F, López-Pajaro LF, et al. Chronic cough in post-COVID syndrome: Laryngeal electromyography findings in vagus nerve neuropathy. PLOS ONE. 30 March 2023;18(3):e0283758.

20. Huang C, Huang L, Wang Y, Li X, Ren L, Gu X, et al. 6-month consequences of COVID-19 in patients discharged from hospital: a cohort study. Lancet Lond Engl. 2021;397(10270):220 32.

21. Arjun MC, Singh AK, Roy P, Ravichandran M, Mandal S, Pal D, et al. Long COVID following Omicron wave in Eastern India-A

retrospective cohort study. J Med Virol. Jan 2023;95(1):e28214.

22. Xiong Q, Xu M, Li J, Liu Y, Zhang J, Xu Y, et al. Clinical sequelae of COVID-19 survivors in Wuhan, China: a single-centre longitudinal study. Clin Microbiol Infect. Jan 2021;27(1):89- 95.

23. Mumtaz A, Sheikh AAE, Khan AM, Khalid SN, Khan J, Nasrullah A, et al. COVID-19 Vaccine and Long COVID: A Scoping Review. Life. 16 Jul 2022;12(7):1066.

24. Yong SJ. Long COVID or post-COVID-19 syndrome: putative pathophysiology, risk factors, and treatments. Infect Dis Lond Engl. 2021:1-18.

25. Munblit D, Bobkova P, Spiridonova E, Shikhaleva A, Gamirova A, Blyuss O, et al. Incidence and risk factors for persistent symptoms in adults previously hospitalized for COVID-.

19. Clin Exp Allergy. Sept 2021;51(9):1107 20.

26. Chelly S, Rouis S, Ezzi O, Ammar A, Fitouri S, Soua A, et al. Symptoms and risk factors for long COVID in Tunisian population. BMC Health Serv Res. 15 May 2023;23:487.

27. Hayat M, Uzair M, Ali Syed R, Arshad M, Bashir S. Status of COVID-19 vaccination around South Asia. Hum Vaccin Immunother. 2022;18(1):2016010.

28. Montani D, Savale L, Noel N, Meyrignac O, Colle R, Gasnier M, et al. Post-acute COVID- 19 syndrome. Eur Respir Rev. 3 March 2022;31(163):210185.

29. Crook H, Raza S, Nowell J, Young M, Edison P. Long covid mechanisms, risk factors, and management. BMJ. 26 Jul 2021;374:n1648.

30. Golchin Vafa R, Heydarzadeh R, Rahmani M, Tavan A, Khoshnoud Mansorkhani S, Zamiri B, et al. The long-term effects of the Covid-19 infection on cardiac symptoms. BMC Cardiovasc Disord. 6 June 2023;23:286.

31. Chopra V, Flanders SA, O'Malley M, Malani AN, Prescott HC. Sixty-Day Outcomes Among Patients Hospitalized With COVID-19. Ann Intern Med. 11 Nov 2020;M20:5661.

32. Alkodaymi MS, Omrani OA, Fawzy NA, Shaar BA, Almamlouk R, Riaz M, et al. Prevalence of post-acute COVID-19 syndrome symptoms at different follow-up periods: a systematic review and meta-analysis. Clin Microbiol Infect. May 2022;28(5):657 66.

33. Mendola M, Leoni M, Cozzi Y, Manzari A, Tonelli F, Metruccio F, et al. Long-term COVID symptoms, work ability and fitness to work in healthcare workers hospitalized for sars-CoV-2 infection.

Med Lav. 2022;113(5):e2022040.

34. Scaramuzzo G, Ronzoni L, Campo G, Priani P, Arena C, La Rosa R, et al. Long-term dyspnea, regional ventilation distribution and peripheral lung function in COVID-19 survivors: a 1 year follow up study. BMC Pulm Med. 9 Nov 2022;22:408.

35. Song WJ, Hui CKM, Hull JH, Birring SS, McGarvey L, Mazzone SB, et al. Confronting COVID-19-associated cough and the post-COVID syndrome: role of viral neurotropism, neuroinflammation, and neuroimmune responses. Lancet Respir Med. May 2021;9(5):533 44.

36. Han X, Fan Y, Alwalid O, Li N, Jia X, Yuan M, et al. Six-Month Follow-up Chest CT findings after Severe COVID-19 Pneumonia. Radiology. apr 2021;299(1):e177-e186.

37. Liu C, Ye L, Xia R, Zheng X, Yuan C, Wang Z, et al. Chest Computed Tomography and Clinical Follow-Up of Discharged Patients with COVID-19 in Wenzhou City, Zhejiang, China. Ann Am Thorac Soc. Oct 2020;17(10):1231.

38. Chilazi M, Duffy EY, Thakkar A, Michos ED. COVID and Cardiovascular Disease: What We Know in 2021. Curr Atheroscler Rep. 2021;23(7):37.

39. Kamal M, Abo Omirah M, Hussein A, Saeed H. Assessment and

characterisation of post- COVID-19 manifestations. Int J Clin Pract. March 2021;75(3):e13746.

40. Davis HE, Assaf GS, McCorkell L, Wei H, Low RJ, Re'em Y, et al. Characterizing long COVID in an international cohort: 7 months of symptoms and their impact. EClinicalMedicine. 15 Jul 2021;38:101019.

41. Huang L, Yao Q, Gu X, Wang Q, Ren L, Wang Y, et al. 1-year outcomes in hospital survivors with COVID-19: a longitudinal cohort study. Lancet Lond Engl. 2021;398(10302):747 58.

42. Brigido S, Manes MT, Ingianni N, Lanni F, Cutolo A, Rovere MTL, et al. Cardiologia di genere: il punto su peculiarità cliniche e fisiopatologiche nelle donne nel long COVID. G Ital Cardiol. 1 Jan 2024;25(1):6 13.

43. Charfeddine S, Ibn Hadj Amor H, Jdidi J, Torjmen S, Kraiem S, Hammami R, et al. Long COVID 19 Syndrome: Is It Related to Microcirculation and Endothelial Dysfunction? Insights From TUN-EndCOV Study. Front Cardiovasc Med. 30 Nov 2021;8:745758.

44. Feter N, Caputo EL, Leite JS, Delpino FM, da Silva LS, Vieira YP, et al. Prevalence and factors associated with long COVID in adults from Southern Brazil: findings from the PAMPA cohort. Cad

Saúde Pública. 2023;39(12):e00098023.

45. Carod-Artal FJ, García-Moncó JC. Epidemiology, pathophysiology, and classification of the neurological symptoms of post-COVID-19 syndrome. Neurol Perspect. Dec 2021;1:S5 15.

46. Williams LD, Zis P. COVID-19-Related Neuropathic Pain: A Systematic Review and Meta- Analysis. J Clin Med. 20 Feb 2023;12(4):1672.

47. Kubota T, Kuroda N, Sone D. Neuropsychiatric aspects of long COVID: A comprehensive review. Psychiatry and Clin Neurosci. Feb 2023;77(2):84-93.

48. Okoye C, Calsolaro V, Calabrese AM, Zotti S, Fedecostante M, Volpato S, et al. Determinants of Cause-Specific Mortality and Loss of Independence in Older Patients following Hospitalization for COVID-19: The GeroCovid Outcomes Study. J Clin Med. 22 Sep 2022;11(19):5578.

49. Hugon J, Queneau M, Sanchez Ortiz M, Msika EF, Farid K, Paquet C. Cognitive decline and brainstem hypometabolism in long COVID: A case series. Brain Behav. 15 March 2022;12(4):e2513.

50. Tana C, Bentivegna E, Cho SJ, Harriott AM, García Azorín D, Labastida-Ramirez A, et al. Long COVID headache. J Headache Pain.

August 1, 2022;23(1):93.

51. Reiter ER, Coelho DH, Kons ZA, Costanzo RM. Subjective smell and taste changes during the COVID-19 pandemic: Short term recovery. Am J Otolaryngol. 2020;41(6):102639.

52. Niklassen AS, Draf J, Huart C, Hintschich C, Bocksberger S, Trecca EMC, et al. COVID - 19: Recovery from Chemosensory Dysfunction. A Multicentre study on Smell and Taste. The Laryngoscope. May 2021;131(5):1095 100.

53. Prem B, Liu DT, Besser G, Sharma G, Dultinger LE, Hofer SV, et al. Long-lasting olfactory dysfunction in COVID-19 patients. Eur Arch Otorhinolaryngol. 2022;279(7):3485 92.

54. Boscolo-Rizzo P, Hummel T, Hopkins C, Dibattista M, Menini A, Spinato G, et al. High prevalence of long-term olfactory, gustatory, and chemesthesis dysfunction in post-COVID-19 patients: a matched case-control study with one-year follow-up using a comprehensive psychophysical evaluation. Rhinology. 1 Dec 2021;59(6):517 27.

55. Kay LM. COVID-19 and olfactory dysfunction: a looming wave of dementia? J Neurophysiol. 1 August 2022;128(2):436 44.

56. Cardoso Soares P, Moreira de Freitas P, de Paula Eduardo C,

Hiramatsu Azevedo L. COVID-19-Related Long-Term Taste Impairment: Symptom Length, Related Taste, Smell Disturbances, and Sample Characteristics. Cureus. Apr 2023;15(4):e38055.

57. Miyazato Y, Tsuzuki S, Morioka S, Terada M, Kutsuna S, Saito S, et al. Factors associated with development and persistence of post-COVID conditions: A cross-sectional study. J Infect Chemother. Sept 2022;28(9):1242 8.

58. Paradowska-Nowakowska E, Łoboda D, Gołba KS, Sarecka-Hujar B. Long COVID-19 Syndrome Severity According to Sex, Time from the Onset of the Disease, and Exercise Capacity-The Results of a Cross-Sectional Study. Life. Feb 2023;13(2):508.

59. Morin L, Savale L, Pham T, Colle R, Figueiredo S, Harrois A, et al. Four-Month Clinical Status of a Cohort of Patients After Hospitalization for COVID-19. JAMA. 20 Apr 2021;325(15):1525 34.

60. Janiri D, Carfì A, Kotzalidis GD, Bernabei R, Landi F, Sani G. Posttraumatic Stress Disorder in Patients After Severe COVID-19 Infection. JAMA Psychiatry. May 2021;78(5):567 9.

61. Mazza MG, Palladini M, De Lorenzo R, Magnaghi C, Poletti S, Furlan R, et al. Persistent psychopathology and neurocognitive impairment in COVID-19 survivors: Effect of inflammatory

biomarkers at three-month follow-up. Brain Behav Immun. May 2021;94:138 47.

62. Fernández-de-las-Peñas C, Gómez-Mayordomo V, de-la-Llave-Rincón AI, Palacios-Ceña M, Rodríguez-Jiménez J, Florencio LL, et al. Anxiety, depression and poor sleep quality as long-term post-COVID sequelae in previously hospitalized patients: A multicenter study. J Infect. Oct 2021;83(4):496 522.

63. Schilling C, Meyer-Lindenberg A, Schweiger JI. Kognitive Störungen und Schlafstörungen bei Long-COVID. Nervenarzt. 2022;93(8):779 87.

64. Ortelli P, Ferrazzoli D, Sebastianelli L, Engl M, Romanello R, Nardone R, et al. Neuropsychological and neurophysiological correlates of fatigue in post-acute patients with neurological manifestations of COVID-19: Insights into a challenging symptom. J Neurol Sci. 15 Jan 2021;420:117271.

65. Ferrandi PJ, Alway SE, Mohamed JS. The interaction between SARS-CoV-2 and ACE2 may have consequences for skeletal muscle viral susceptibility and myopathies. J Appl Physiol. 1 Oct 2020;129(4):864 7.

66. Karaarslan F, Güneri FD, Kardeş S. Long COVID:

rheumatologic/musculoskeletal symptoms in hospitalized COVID-19 survivors at 3 and 6 months. Clin Rheumatol. 2022;41(1):289 96.

67. Aiyegbusi OL, Hughes SE, Turner G, Rivera SC, McMullan C, Chandan JS, et al. Symptoms, complications and management of long COVID: a review. J R Soc Med. Sept 2021;114(9):428 42.

68. Carvalho-Schneider C, Laurent E, Lemaignen A, Beaufils E, Bourbao-Tournois C, Laribi S, et al. Follow-up of adults with noncritical COVID-19 two months after symptom onset. Clin Microbiol Infect. Feb 2021;27(2):258 63.

69. Lauwers M, Au M, Yuan S, Wen C. COVID-19 in Joint Ageing and Osteoarthritis: Current Status and Perspectives. Int J Mol Sci. 10 Jan 2022;23(2):720.

70. Loosen SH, Jensen BEO, Tanislav C, Luedde T, Roderburg C, Kostev K. Obesity and lipid metabolism disorders determine the risk for development of long COVID syndrome: a cross-sectional study from 50,402 COVID-19 patients. Infection. 2022;50(5):1165 70.

71. Nabavi N. Long covid: How to define it and how to manage it. BMJ. 7 Sep 2020;370:m3489.

72. Fatima G, Bhatt D, Idrees J, Khalid B, Mahdi F. Elucidating Post-COVID-19 manifestations in India. BMJ. 2021;1-12.

73. Magnusson K, Kristoffersen DT, Dell'Isola A, Kiadaliri A, Turkiewicz A, Runhaar J, et al. Post-covid medical complaints following infection with SARS-CoV-2 Omicron vs Delta variants. Nat Commun. 30 Nov 2022;13(1):7363.

74. Antonelli M, Pujol JC, Spector TD, Ourselin S, Steves CJ. Risk of long COVID associated with delta versus omicron variants of SARS-CoV-2. The Lancet. June 2022;399(10343):2263 4.

75. Fernández-de-las-Peñas C, Torres-Macho J, Velasco-Arribas M, Arias-Navalón JA, Guijarro C, Hernández-Barrera V, et al. Similar prevalence of long-term post-COVID symptoms in patients with asthma: A case-control study. The Journal of Infection. August 2021;83(2):237.

76. Garcia-Pachon E, Grau-Delgado J, Soler-Sempere MJ, Zamora-Molina L, Baeza-Martinez C, Ruiz-Alcaraz S, et al. Low prevalence of post-COVID-19 syndrome in patients with asthma. J Infect. June 2021;82(6):276 316.

77. Chen Y, Zhang X, Zeng X, Xu T, Xiao W, Yang X, et al. Prevalence and risk factors for postinfectious cough in discharged patients with coronavirus disease 2019 (COVID-19). J Thorac Dis. June 2022;14(6):2079 88.

78. Islam MdK, Hossain MF, Molla MdMA, Sharif MdM, Hasan P, Hossain FS, et al. A 2- month post-COVID-19 follow-up study on patients with dyspnea. Health Sci Rep. 17 Nov 2021;4(4):e435.

79. Garcia-Azorin D, Layos-Romero A, Porta-Etessam J, Membrilla JA, Caronna E, Gonzalez- Martinez A, et al. Post-COVID-19 persistent headache: A multicentric 9-months follow-up study of 905 patients. Cephalalgia. Jul 2022;42(8):804 9.

80. Romero-Rodríguez E, Pérula-de Torres LÁ, Castro-Jiménez R, González-Lama J, Jiménez- García C, González-Bernal JJ, et al. Hospital admission and vaccination as predictive factors of long COVID-19 symptoms. Front Med. 11 Nov 2022;9:1016013.

81. Mińko A, Turoń-Skrzypińska A, Rył A, Tomska N, Bereda Z, Rotter I. Searching for Factors Influencing the Severity of the Symptoms of Long COVID. Int J Environ Res Public Health. 30 June 2022;19(13):8013.

82. Badenoch JB, Rengasamy ER, Watson C, Jansen K, Chakraborty S, Sundaram RD, et al. Persistent neuropsychiatric symptoms after COVID-19: a systematic review and meta-analysis. Brain Commun. 17 Dec 2021;4(1):fcab297.

83. Zhang X, Wang F, Shen Y, Zhang X, Cen Y, Wang B, et al.

Symptoms and Health Outcomes Among Survivors of COVID-19 Infection 1 Year After Discharge From Hospitals in Wuhan, China. JAMA Netw Open. 29 Sep 2021;4(9):e2127403.

84. Kaur D, Agrawal KC, Deep A, Choudhary H, Soni L, Saran R, et al. Post-COVID-19 manifestations: A study of analyzing symptoms, complications following hospitalization. J Fam Med Prim Care. Oct 2022;11(10):6015 22.

85. Swarnakar R, Jenifa S, Wadhwa S. Musculoskeletal complications in long COVID-19: A systematic review. World J Virol. 25 Nov 2022;11(6):485 95.

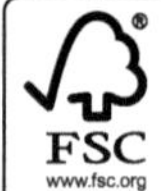

MIX
Papier aus verantwortungsvollen Quellen
Paper from responsible sources
FSC® C105338

Printed by Books on Demand GmbH, Norderstedt / Germany